NOV   2005

McGovern School Library
9 Lovering Street
Medway, MA 02053

W9-BFA-246

The Library of Healthy Living™

Staying Healthy:

Dental Care

Alice B. McGinty

The Rosen Publishing Group's
PowerKids Press™
New York

Published in 1997 by The Rosen Publishing Group, Inc.
29 East 21st Street, New York, NY 10010

Copyright © 1997 by The Rosen Publishing Group, Inc.

All rights reserved. No part of this book may be reproduced in any form without permission in writing from the publisher, except by a reviewer.

First Edition

Book Design: Kim Sonsky

Photo Credits: Cover by Seth Dinnerman; p. 9 © Arthur Tilley/FPG International; p. 10 © Bill Losh/FPG International; all photo illustrations by Seth Dinnerman.

McGinty, Alice B.
      Staying healthy: Dental care / Alice B. McGinty.
            p.   cm. (The library of healthy living)
      Summary: Provides an overview of the teeth, including the different kinds of teeth we have, their composition, and how to take care of them.
      ISBN 0-8239-5139-1
      1. Dental care—Juvenile literature. 2. Teeth—Juvenile literature. [1. Teeth. 2. Dental care.]
I. Title. II. Series.
RK63.M39 1997
617.6'01—dc21   96-37360
                                                                                              CIP
                                                                                               AC

Manufactured in the United States of America

Contents

Your Terrific Teeth

Your teeth do great things for you. They brighten your smile. They help you eat. They even help you speak.

Say the word "tooth." Your tongue touches your front teeth to make the "th" sound. Without your teeth there, the word "tooth" would sound funny.

Your teeth and **gums** (GUMZ) need special care to stay healthy. Your teeth are an important part of your body. Take care of them and they will keep doing great things for you.

Your teeth and gums also help to give your face its nice, round shape. ▶

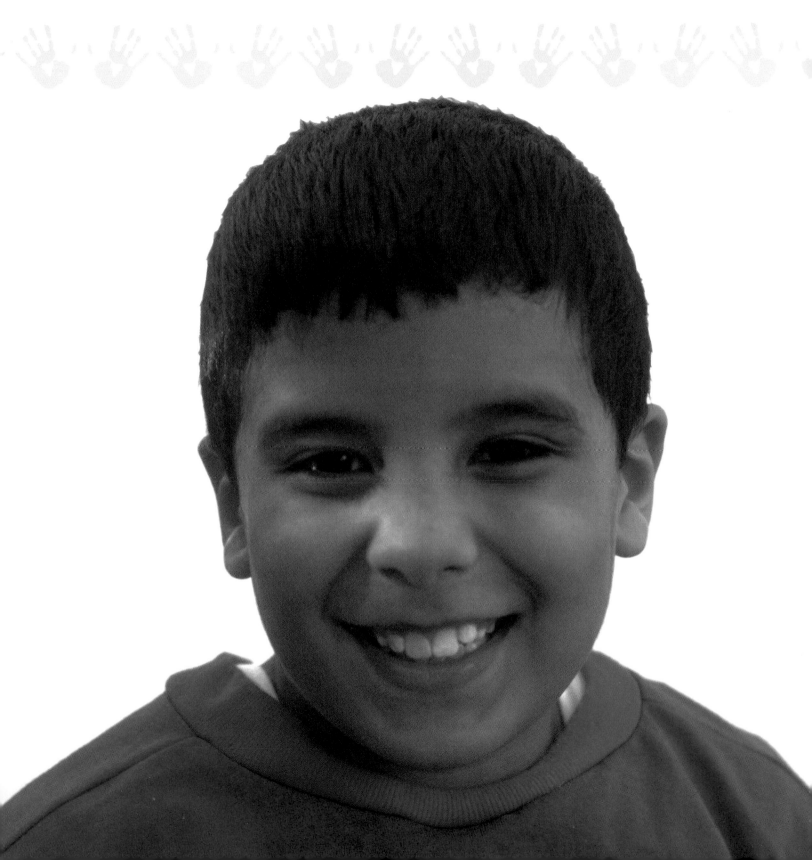

Different Teeth for Different Jobs

You have different kinds of teeth that do different jobs.

Your front teeth are called **incisors** (in-SY-zerz). Their job is to bite. Their wide, sharp tops can bite through a crisp apple or a crunchy carrot.

Your pointy teeth are called **canines** (KAY-nynz), or **cuspids** (KUS-pidz). Their job is to tear foods. They are called "canines" after dogs, whose pointed teeth can tear meat.

The big, flat teeth in the back of your mouth are called **molars** (MOH-lerz). Their job is to chew.

You have eight incisors, four canines, and eight molars. ▶

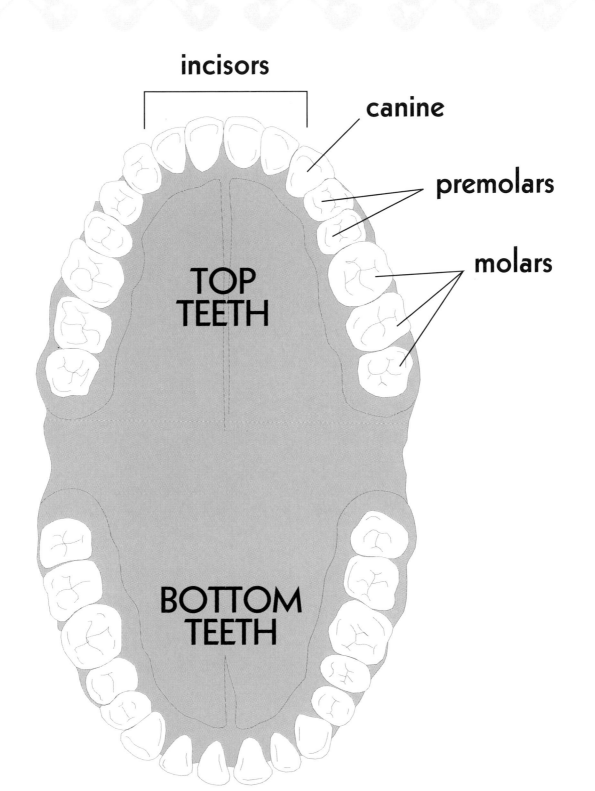

incisors

canine

premolars

molars

TOP
TEETH

BOTTOM
TEETH

Your Primary Teeth

When you were born, you probably had no teeth. Your teeth were still growing inside your gums. Then, when they were ready, your teeth pushed up through your gums one by one.

You probably got your first tooth when you were about six months old. Then more teeth came. By the time you were around two years old, you had twenty teeth in your mouth. Those twenty teeth are called **primary** (PRY-mayr-ee) teeth.

Primary teeth are also known as baby teeth. ▶

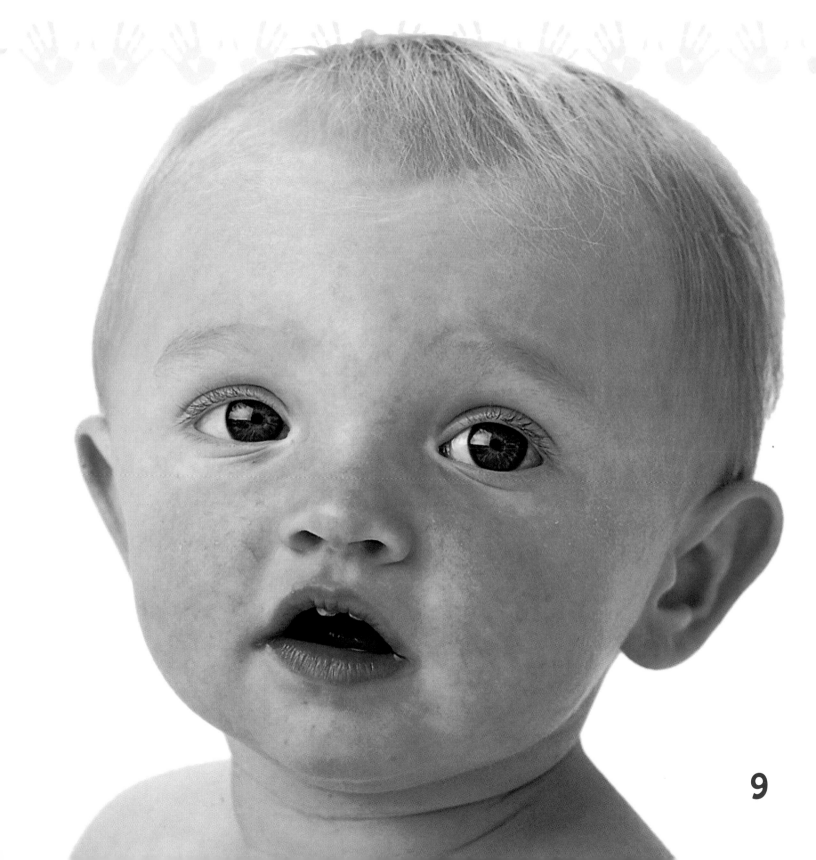

9

Losing Your Primary Teeth

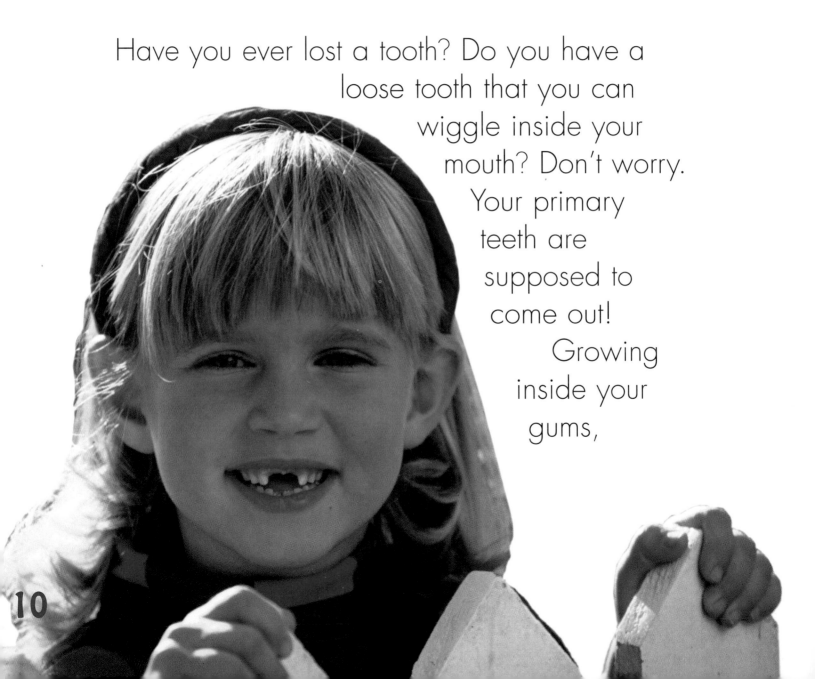

Have you ever lost a tooth? Do you have a loose tooth that you can wiggle inside your mouth? Don't worry. Your primary teeth are supposed to come out! Growing inside your gums,

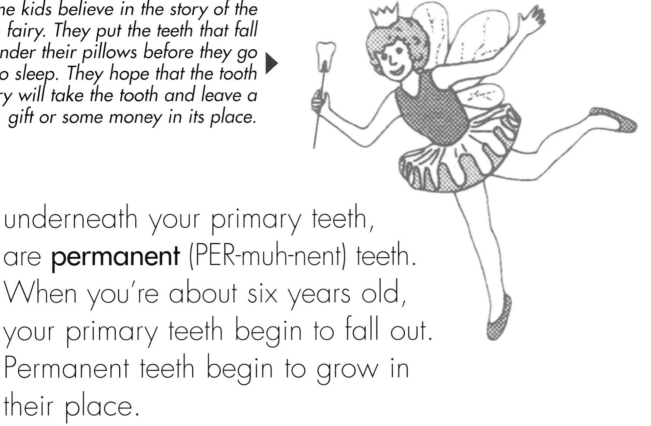

Some kids believe in the story of the tooth fairy. They put the teeth that fall out under their pillows before they go to sleep. They hope that the tooth fairy will take the tooth and leave a gift or some money in its place.

underneath your primary teeth, are **permanent** (PER-muh-nent) teeth. When you're about six years old, your primary teeth begin to fall out. Permanent teeth begin to grow in their place.

Now that your mouth has grown bigger, you have room for your permanent teeth. These are the teeth you will have for the rest of your life.

11

Your Permanent Teeth

PREMOLAR

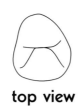

front view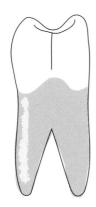

top view

The first permanent teeth that grow in are called premolars, or baby molars. A set of permanent molars grows in behind your premolars.

Then come your incisors. Sometimes permanent incisors are bumpy on top because the teeth have grown faster in some places than others. In time, they will become smooth.

INCISOR

front view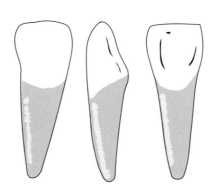

back view

side view

CANINE

side view 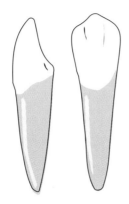 back view

Next, the **bicuspids** (by-KUS-pidz), canines, and second molars grow in.

By the time you're twelve years old, you should have 28 permanent teeth. Four molars, called **wisdom** (WIZ-dum) teeth, will grow in later to make a full set. That's 32 teeth!

MOLAR

front view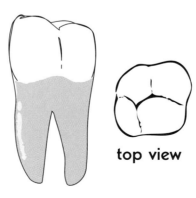

top view

A Closer Look at Your Teeth

When you look at a tooth, you see its **crown** (KROWN). The outside of the crown is made of **enamel** (ee-NAM-ul). Enamel is harder than anything else in your body. It protects the tooth and stays strong through lots of chewing.

Underneath the enamel is hard, bone-like **dentin** (DEN-tin).

In the center of the tooth is soft **pulp** (PULP).

Underneath your gums is the **root** (ROOT) of the tooth. The root carries blood and **nerves** (NERVZ) into the pulp. Nerves sense heat, cold, and pain.

A Healthy Tooth

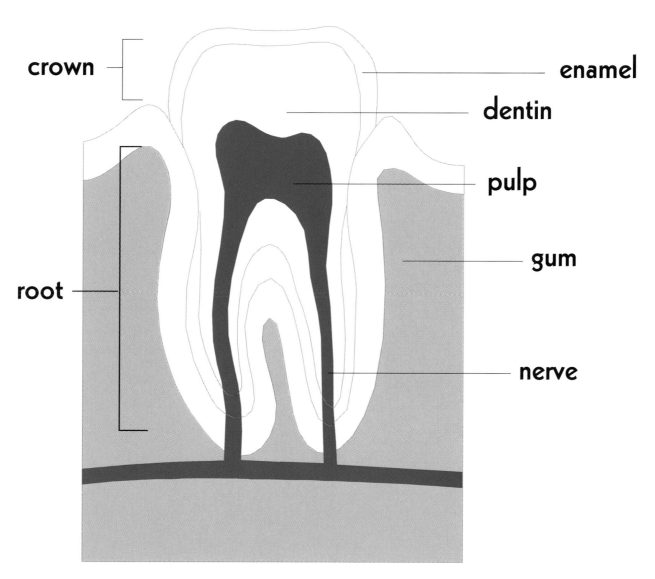

crown

enamel

dentin

pulp

gum

root

nerve

15

Tooth Decay

Although teeth are hard, some things can hurt them.

Tiny **bacteria** (bak-TEER-ee-uh) live in parts of your mouth. They can stick to your teeth to make a clear, sticky film called **plaque** (PLAK). Dental plaque that gets hard is called tartar. Tartar can hurt your gums.

The sugar from foods you eat or things that you drink sticks to the plaque and makes **acid** (A-sid). Acid hurts teeth by eating away the enamel. If acid stays on the tooth too long, it can make a hole, or **cavity** (KAV-ih-tee).

When acid eats away at the enamel, it is called tooth **decay** (dee-KAY).

A Tooth with Cavities

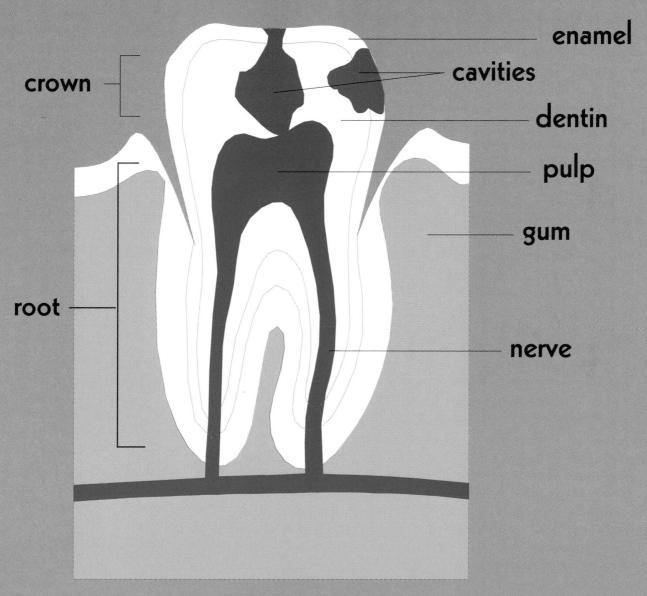

enamel

cavities

dentin

pulp

gum

nerve

crown

root

Brush and Floss!

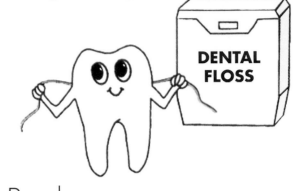

DENTAL FLOSS

What can you do to protect your teeth from decay?

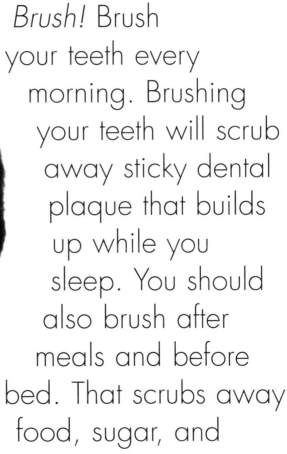

Brush! Brush your teeth every morning. Brushing your teeth will scrub away sticky dental plaque that builds up while you sleep. You should also brush after meals and before bed. That scrubs away food, sugar, and

18

acid. Brush the front, back, sides, and tops of your teeth. Gently brush your gums too.

Floss! Dental floss is a waxy thread. You pull it between your teeth before or after you brush them to get rid of food and plaque from between teeth and on your gums. Flossing is important because it reaches places that your toothbrush can't. It's a good idea to floss every day.

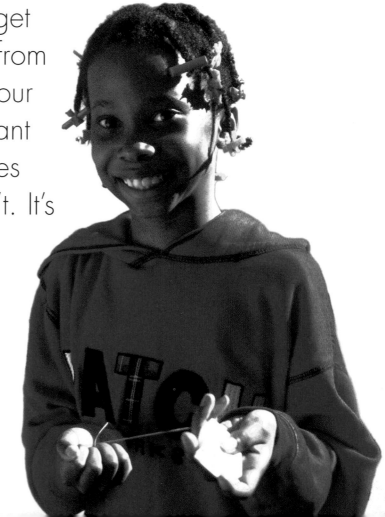

Sugar

Many foods have sugar inside them—even foods that don't taste sweet, like crackers. Each time you eat these foods, your teeth are covered with sugar. The longer sugar stays on your teeth, the more chances there are for it to make tooth-decaying acid. Sticky sugars, such as gum or caramel, stay on your teeth even longer. What can you do? Eat sugar less often, or with meals. Brush your teeth after you eat. If you can't brush, drink water to rinse your teeth.

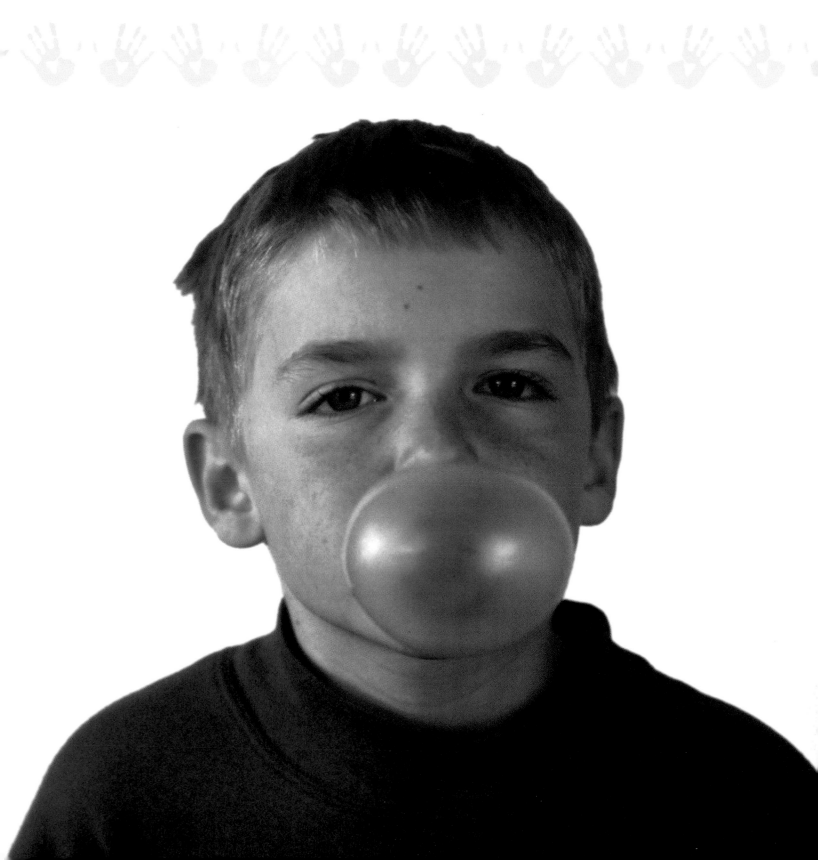

Taking Care of Your Teeth

There are many ways for you to take care of your teeth.

☺ Use toothpaste with **fluoride** (FLOOR-yd). Fluoride makes your teeth harder and stronger.

☺ Visit your dentist at least twice a year. Your dentist will clean your teeth, give your teeth a fluoride treatment, and check for tooth decay. If you have a cavity, the dentist will clean and fill it so it will not get bigger.

Take good care of your teeth. They are an important part of a strong, healthy you!

Glossary

acid (A-sid) A tooth-decaying substance made from bacteria and sugar.

bacteria (bak-TEER-ee-uh) Tiny living things that sometimes cause illness or decay.

bicuspid (by-KUS-pid) A molar with two points.

canine tooth (KAY-nyn TOOTH) A pointed tooth. It is also called a cuspid.

cavity (KAV-ih-tee) A soft spot or hole in a tooth.

crown (KROWN) The top part of a tooth.

cuspid (KUS-pid) A pointed tooth. It is also called a canine tooth.

decay (dee-KAY) When acid eats away at a tooth and hurts it.

dentin (DEN-tin) The bone-like part of the tooth under the enamel.

enamel (ee-NAM-ul) The hard covering of the crown of the tooth.

fluoride (FLOOR-yd) A substance that makes teeth harder and stronger.

gum (GUM) The flesh around teeth.

incisor (in-SY-zer) A wide, sharp front tooth.

molar (MOH-ler) A big, flat back tooth.

nerve (NERV) Part of the body that feels heat, cold, and pain.

permanent tooth (PER-muh-nent TOOTH) An adult tooth.

plaque (PLAK) A clear, sticky film made when bacteria sticks to teeth.

primary tooth (PRY-mayr-ee TOOTH) A baby tooth.

pulp (PULP) The soft center of a tooth.

root (ROOT) The part of the tooth underneath the gum.

wisdom tooth (WIZ-dum TOOTH) A permanent molar that grows in last.

Index